SPRINGS OF LIFE

Spring To Life

VEVINE GOLDSON

DEDICATION

This book is dedicated to natural healing and nature's medicine.

TABLE OF CONTENTS

INTRODUCTION

Do not underestimate the power of plants:Many people from ancient times Throughout the Caribbean Africa Asia And Europe has been using plants herbs shrubs wild weed to feed themselves and cure many ailments and illnesses,and even today some of these practices still live on.

Take for instances in the caribbean deep in the villages that have no shops nor doctors nearby,they depend on the greens and wild weeds of the earth to raise them and their children and not surprisingly a lot of them live straight up until they reach 90 even 100 years old;So do not underestimate the healing properties of plants.
Plants are power packed with nutrients and has a number of healing properties that can keep our immune system working in good condition,and scientists around the world are catching on.

1/   SARSAPILLA WEED

This wild weed is grown all over the deep forests of Jamaica and is known as cocolmeca,and belong to the smilax genus family. Harvested for its medicinal properties and is used to treat a number of conditions,such as blood clots skin irritations,joint pains,headaches,leprosy,arthritis,common colds,sexual impotence,psoriasis,rheumatoid,anemia,STDS, herpese.

In 1889 the sarsapilla weed was researched by a doctor known as Charles E Hires and he found that it had a certain property that can be used in soft drinks and beer.

The fever grass is a weed that is grown and harvested throughout jamaica,for its sweet minty aroma and healing properties. The other name for this weed is lemon grass. It is grown upwards and has long thin green leaves that are easy to harvest. It's commonly taken as a tea but can be brewed into a cold summer drink some have theirs with a dash of rum.
It is said to have natural anti-inflammatory properties,anti-cancer,is used to treat kidney problems,and with its sweet minty taste is used to flavour meats and cakes,brewed and taken as a tonic and is used as air vaporizer and essential oil.

CERASEE

The cerasee plant is grown harvested and sold all over Jamaica;Though a native to the caribbean it can be found in other parts of the world. The other name for the cerasee is marmadica charantia.
The plant is easily identified because it grows a yellow fruit called bitter guard or bitter melon,the yellow fruit can be eaten raw and is used to flavour dishes cakes meats and puddings. The leaves are boild and is used to treat parasitic worms,common ailments like hypertension,diabetes,urinary tract infection,skin inflammations,purging of the blood and kidneys.
It has vitamin A C and iron.

The leaf of life is common in Jamaica,it's also known as Bryophyllum;It's used throughout the world for its medicine and in Jamaica it's used to treat all kinds of ailments. Other common names are love bush,wonder of the world,miracle leaf and live forever.
The best thing is its liver healing properties,it is anti-fungal,antiviral,anti-bacterial.
I use to eat it raw when I was a child,I would pick the leaves wash them and chew them raw with sugar.
You can boil it in a brew drink as tonic,squeeze the juices over cuts and grazes and use in the ear to help speed up the healing process if there's an infection.

The wisdom weed has many names such as ganja,marijuana,canabis weed and many more. The rastas call it the wisdom weed according to their doctrine it's a sacred weed that gives them enlightenment and wisdom. Around the world people that follow the Jamaican rasta religion and party goers smoke this weed for its calming effect. The rastas in Jamaica has been using it for many years for its spiritual and healing properties and the world has caught on;Despite the many back-lashings the jamaican rastas and their followers did not give up on the holy weed,and now doctors around the world has started to acknoweledge that it is indeed a medicine.California was the first state to legalise it in 1996. It's used to flavour dishes and cakes,cure ailments,inhale as a vaporIzor and many more.

Jack in the bush is a wild invasive weed that grows in the wild forests of Jamaica. It is known scientifically as Eupatorium Odoratum,and it's a very popular medicinal herb in certain parishes of jamaica. Other common names are christmas bush,siam weed,bitter bush,agrimony and hemp.
It's medicinal and is used to treat people that are suffering from bronchiatists,asma,and many different skin inflammations;Other illnesses that it's used to treat are diabetes,sinusitis,fever common colds and flu.

 SPIRIT WEED

The spirit weed is a common and wild invasive weed that grows throughout jamaica's forests plains and deep woods.The scientific name for it is Eryngium Foetidum;It's used to flavour dishes taken as tonic and drink as tea.
Other common names are shadon,fit weed and spirit,the stems root and leaves are used for various dishes and flavourings,but most times it is harvested because of its medicinal properties.
It's used as an essential oil in baths and as an air vaporizer. It's used to cure fever heal wounds kill parasitic worms,cure snake and scorpian bites,ease blood pressure,epilepsy and diarrhea.
It's packed with iron riboflavin protein and vitamins such as vitamin A B1 B2 and C.

The spanish needle is a pretty looking wild herb that can be found growing in the deep forest of jamaica. It's easily seen because of its bright white petals and yellow blooms. Other common names are black jack,cobblers peg,ghost needle weed,demon spike grass,beggars tick,needle grass and broom tick.
It has medicinal properties that are used to treat diabetes,bronchitis,bacterial infections,hepatitis,asma,urinary tract infection,colds flu,and it help to speed up the healing process of cuts and deep wounds.

9/ PERIWINKLE

The periwinkle is a common and wild weed that is grown in the deep forest and garden of jamaica. It is commonly known as ram goat roses creeping myrtle and vinca.
It's an invasive weed but is also harvested around the caribbean and other parts of the world for its medicinal properties;The herb can be used internally and externally,for common illnesses such as heavy menstrual bleeding,gastritis,diarrhea.
It's used to speed up the health of the mucous membrane,and is also used as an anticeptic agent to cure throat infections,gingivitis and mouth ulcers.
The medicinal property in periwinkle is called vincamine.

Search mi heart is a wild invasive weed that can be found growing in the forests and gardens of many jamaicans. Other common names for this weed is search my heart,search me heart;According to researches that had been carried out it can only be found in jamaica,but not sure if that's still the same. This common weed is connected to many folk stories in the caribbean carried on from many generations as far back as the 1800.
It's harvested for its medicinal properties that is mainly used in the treatment of speeding up the healing process of heart troubles,hence the name.
It's brewed and taken as a tonic for its anti-inflammatory and anti-bacterial healing,it's also used as an antioxidant.

The soursop tree is a fruit plant that can be found commonly growing in the garden and wild of jamaica,and many parts of the world. Scientifically it's known as Annonamuricata and the active compound in its plant is called Annaceousacetogenins;Both the leaves and the fruit is power packed with nutrients and healing properties.
It's rich in vitamins A B and C and has an acid called gentillic acid.
It is used in to flavour many culinary dishes used as spice for meats and baked goods. The fruit when juiced is milky white and thick and is used to compliment sunday dinners in the caribbean.
It is known throughout the world for its strong anti-cancer properties,but it's also used to treat rhoumatism,gout,diabetes,depression. It also heals ulcers and helps to repair organs.

The guinea hen weed is widely spread in the back bushes and gardens of the caribbean especially jamaica. It's wild and is known to be very invasive but it's harvested because of medicinal properties. The scientific name for it is Phytolaccaceae.
The plant has a very strong odour similar to garlic and when animals graze it as a food source,it gives off a very strong smell in the milk and meat. It's anti-inflammatory,anti-bacterial,and can be used as a sedative;It also has anti-cancer properties.
Scientists have discovered its biological active compound and now more researches are being done.
It's very rich in vitamins and minerals.

The Joseph's coat plant is a flower that spreads like the sun with its colourful leaves that springs out all around its stalk. It has become one of national treasure and has been germinated for medicine and decoration.
Its name derive from a holy book that refers to the coat given to joseph in biblical times that has many different colours. The plant is a heat lover so it thrives in the tropics and anywhere where it's warm;Easy to recognize with its beautiful array of bright wine and green yellow leaves;The josephs coat is power packed with vitamins and minerals and some countries that are aware of this use it to make salads and grind the seeds to make flour.
The caribbean folks drink it as a brew for its anti-fungal anti-bacteria healing properties.
It has many other healing uses and is said to be one of the most in demand botanical plant.

Eventhough herbs are use to heal a number of ailments and illnesses;You must never go about it without seeking the advise of an expert for proper dosage.

Healing with herbs have been around from ancient times.

Herbs plants shrubs is known as nature's medicine, they can help us to reconnect with our own spirituality.

ABOUT THE AUTHOR

Vevine Goldson likes to promote healthy lifestyles.
Check her other books for more on healthy living. (The Book Of Life) (Beauty Face Mask For Women And Men) (Therapeutic And Yummy Spa Tips From Home).